YOUR KNOWLEDGE HAS VALUE

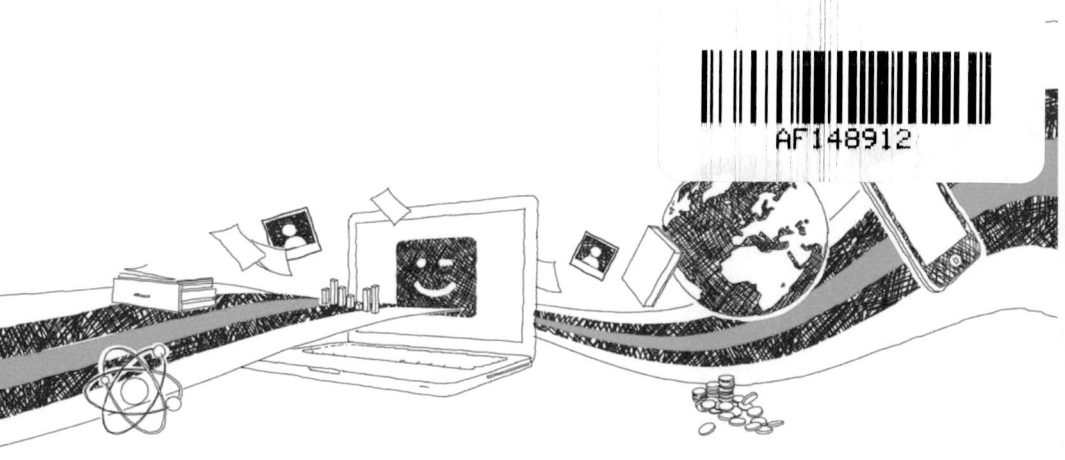
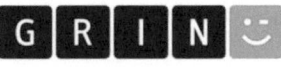

Don Johnson Villanueva

Anti-Thrombocytopenic and Hemostatic Effect of Papaya (Carica papaya) on Aspirin Induced-ICR Mice

A Screening for Anti-Dengue Property

GRIN Publishing

Bibliographic information published by the German National Library:

The German National Library lists this publication in the National Bibliography; detailed bibliographic data are available on the Internet at http://dnb.dnb.de .

Imprint:

Copyright © 2014 GRIN Verlag GmbH
Print and binding: Books on Demand GmbH, Norderstedt Germany
ISBN: 978-3-656-95774-4

This book at GRIN:

http://www.grin.com/en/e-book/299211/anti-thrombocytopenic-and-hemostatic-effect-of-papaya-carica-papaya-on

GRIN - Your knowledge has value

Since its foundation in 1998, GRIN has specialized in publishing academic texts by students, college teachers and other academics as e-book and printed book. The website www.grin.com is an ideal platform for presenting term papers, final papers, scientific essays, dissertations and specialist books.

Visit us on the internet:

http://www.grin.com/

http://www.facebook.com/grincom

http://www.twitter.com/grin_com

Anti-Thrombocytopenic and Hemostatic Effect of Papaya (*Carica papaya*) on Aspirin Induced- ICR Mice: A Screening for Anti-Dengue Property

DON JOHNSON MIRANDA VILLANUEVA
Maria Victoria D. Tuazon, RMT, MPH

ABSTRACT

Aims: To investigate the Anti-thrombocytopenic and Hemostatic effect of Papaya fresh fruit extract in the sub-normal platelet counts and other blood components of ICR mice induced by Aspirin.
Study design: *In vivo* biological assay.
Place and Duration of Study: Zoology Laboratory, Biology Department, College of Science, Bicol University, Legazpi City, between October and November 2013.
Methodology: Mice were induced with Aspirin and treated with varying concentrations of Papaya fruit extract: Low, Medium and High, including the Negative and Positive controls with three replicates each. Blood samples were collected through tail vein method on day 0, seventh day and fourteenth day. Automated CBC, determination of bleeding time and clotting time, and weighing were also completed on the abovementioned days to attain the required data.
Results: In terms of platelet count, significant differences among the treatments were found by ANOVA during the 7th and 14th day of treatment (p=0.000). In terms of clotting time, it only took a week for all the treatment groups to shorten the clotting time as compared to the positive control. However, the low and medium concentration extract-treated groups manifested better results on the second week. RBC counts differed significantly among treatments on the 7th day. Weight of all test animals increased (p=0.012) during the 7th day. A gain in weight of the animals treated with varying concentrations was also observed during the 14th day of administration (p=0.000).
Conclusion: The results suggest that the use of Papaya fruit extract may be beneficial in treating the adverse effect of Dengue virus- thrombocytopenia.

Keywords: Carica papaya, Dengue virus, Thrombocytopenia, Anti-thrombocytopenia, Hemostatic

1. INTRODUCTION

The feared disease, dengue, has been touching significant prevalent levels with numerous records of patients infected and with its increasing death toll unchanged, it has formed a nationwide crisis. A remedy for this dreaded disease however is still in wanting and it has now become a major international public health problem. Dengue Hemorrhagic Fever (DHF), as it's medically known, is a potentially fatal complication, resulting in bleeding and thrombocytopenia where there is an abnormally low level of blood platelets in the body. Platelets play an essential physiological role in blood coagulation (Gregg and Clermont, 2003). Dengue as a disease caused by the bite of *Aedes aegypti* mosquito was first recognized during dengue epidemics in the Philippines and Thailand in the 1950s (WHO, 1997). The symptoms of dengue include high-grade fever, rashes, and severe headache. Additional manifestations include severe joint and muscle pain, loss of appetite, vomiting, and eye pain. Dengue fever itself is fatal, or it can be an extraordinarily painful and disabling illness and may become epidemic in a population following the introduction of a new serotype (Knowlton, 2009).

Millions of people in several traditional schemes have resorted to the use of medicinal plants to treat their ailments, and this could be a result either of the high cost of established health care or low supply of available medication. In this light, it is a great concern to the researcher that other plants can be also examined to determine if they improve one's health or well-being. In the study at hand, the researcher would like to focus on the use of Papaya fruit, in its fresh form, on thrombocytes of albino mice.

Papaya, scientifically known as *Carica papaya,* is a perennial plant and is presently distributed over the whole tropical regions and has spread over many other sub-tropical countries including the Philippines. In the field of medicine, it is traditionally used to treat indigestion and have also been shown to possess other curative effects.

The general objective of this study is to screen the Anti-Dengue and Hemostatic properties of Papaya fruit extract on ICR mice. Specifically, the study aimed to achieve the following objectives: first, to determine the anti-thrombocytopenic effect on platelet count of mice; second: to determine its hemostatic effect in bleeding time and blood-clotting time; third: to observe if the extract would also affect the number of red blood cells and white blood cells of mice; and lastly, to determine if the extract would affect the weight of mice.

2. MATERIALS AND METHODS

2.1 Preparation of the fruit extract

A fresh ripe fruit of *Carica papaya* was collected at Bicol University College of Agriculture and Forestry, Guinobatan, Albay and brought immediately by the researcher to Bicol University College of Science, Legazpi City for extraction. The fresh fruit weighing 1kg was washed thoroughly with tap water, and wiped with clean cloth for drying. It was peeled and sliced into half. The seeds were removed from the center of the fruit using a large spoon and the flesh was further sliced into smaller pieces and was blended. The fruit extract was filtered using cheese cloth to separate the residues from the extract. The filtration was repeated until no solid residues were visible. Preparation of different concentrations of the extract was done immediately after the extraction.

2.2 Treatment preparation

Three different concentrations were prepared for the treatment. The low concentration was composed of 25% of the prepared extract and 75% of distilled water. For medium concentration, it was composed of 50% extract and 50% of distilled water and for the high concentration, 75% of extract and 25% of distilled water. The mixtures were stored separately in sterilized glass bottles and refrigerated prior to use.

2.3 Experimental Animals

A total of thirty (30) male Imprinting Control Region (ICR) laboratory albino mice (*Mus musculus*) of 7 weeks old, weighing within the range of 20 to 25 g were purchased from the Bureau of Animal Industry, Diliman, Quezon City.

2.4 Induction of Thrombocytopenia

Two hundred and fifty milligrams (250 mg) of Acetylsalicylic Acid (Aspirin) was dissolved in 10mL of distilled water to give a concentration of 25 mg/mL. The dosage of aspirin administration in this study was accorded from the protocol of Chaloob *et. al.* (2009). The induction was performed through oral administration and platelet count of each animal was observed 24 hours after administration.

2.5 Experimental Design

After acclimatization and induction of thrombocytopenia, mice were weighed randomly divided into the following groups. All animals were fed with their regular diet of mice pellets and distilled water *ad libitum* for 14 days.

T_0R_2	T_2R_3	T_0R_1	T_0R_3	T_3R_2
T_1R_3	T_1R_1	T_3R_3	T_4R_1	T_3R_1
T_2R_2	T_4R_2	T_4R_3	T_2R_1	T_1R_2

Figure 1. Bioassay experimental design

Treatment		Replicate	
T0	Negative Control (Distilled H20)	R1	Replicate 1
T1	Low Concentration (25% papaya fruit extract + 75% H20 + Aspirin Induced)	R2	Replicate 2
T2	Low Concentration (50% papaya fruit extract + 50% H20 + Aspirin Induced)	R3	Replicate 3
T3	High Concentration (75% papaya fruit extract + 25% H20 + Aspirin Induced)	R4	Replicate 4
T4	Positive Control (Aspirin Induced)	R5	Replicate 5

2.6. Determination of Weight

Animals were weighed before (Day 0), on the seventh day, and after the period of administration (Day 14). Same time of weighing were strictly observed and proper tagging was used for accurate identification purposes. Complete blood count including Platelet count, bleeding time and blood-clotting time was also monitored before the introduction of the treatment (time-zero samples), on the seventh day and after the 14-day administration of the extract, by collecting tail blood samples from the mice.

2.7 Determination of Platelet, Red Blood Cell and White Blood Cell Counts

Blood was collected via the tail vein method. In this procedure, the mouse was retrained with the tail exposed. The tip of the tail was warmed using hot compress cleaned with alcohol. With the tail under gentle traction, and the needle at a very shallow angle to the tail, the needle was inserted into the lumen of the lateral tail vein, which lies immediately beneath the skin on each side of the tail. Collected tail blood samples (0.5 mL) were placed on EDTA bottles and analyzed on Ago General Hospital Laboratory Department using Mindray Automated Hematology Analyzer for complete blood count to establish required data.

2.8 Determination of Bleeding time

Bleeding time was determined using Duke's method with some modifications. The tail was cleaned with warm distilled water and sterile gauze. Venipuncture on the tail was done by using a lancelet. Biopette micropipette was used to collect 0.5 mL of blood from the exposed bleeding tail and transferred on a glass slide. The collected blood was blotted on a No. 9 Whatman filter paper. The time from first application to the disappearance of blood was recorded. This procedure was repeated during every blood collection.

2.9 Determination of Blood-clotting time

Blood clotting time measurement method to be used in this study is adapted from the study of Apostol, et, al., (2013). The tail was also cleaned with warm distilled water and sterile gauze. Puncture on the tail vein was done by using a lancelet. Biopette micropipette was used to collect 1 mL of blood from the exposed bleeding tail and transferred on a glass slide. The blood drop on the glass slide was rubbed using a lancet until fibrin threads were seen. The time from first contact with lancet and the formation of threads was recorded. Same procedure was repeated during every blood collection.

2.3.0 Statistical Analysis

The data gathered were analyzed using Analysis of Variance (ANOVA) to determine the significant differences among treatments. Duncan's Multiple Range Test (DMRT) was also used as a post-hoc procedure, to determine if there exist significant differences in the treatment groups during the course of the treatment phase.

3. RESULTS AND DISCUSSIONS

3.1 Effect on Platelet count

Platelet counts of mice significantly decreased after induction with Acetylsalicylic acid (Aspirin). Imitating the main effect of dengue virus, this decrease in platelet count corresponds to the altered platelet distribution by the drug which is responsible for the development of thrombocytopenia as stated by Botting (2006). Aspirin's ability to suppress the production prostaglandins and thromboxanes is due to its irreversible inactivation of the cyclooxygenase (COX) enzyme (Botting, 2006). Platelet cyclooxygenase or prostaglandin synthase is the target of several anti-platelet agents, like Aspirin, than can block the activity of the enzyme by competing with the substrate or permanently altering active sites, respectively.

In regard to platelet count (Figure 2), ANOVA revealed significant differences among the treatments during the 7th and 14th day of treatment (p=0.000). Platelet counts of untreated mice decreased after the induction of Aspirin.

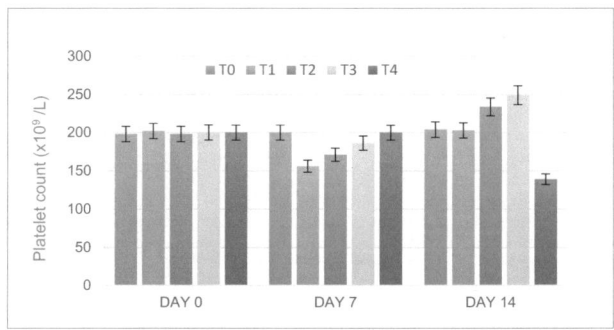

Figure 2. Platelet count of mice at varying concentrations of *Carica papaya* fruit extract

The study showed that after the induction of thrombocytopenia, there is a significant differences among the treatments during the 7th and 14th day of treatment (p=0.000). This illustrates that the varying concentrations of the extracts are effective in treating the said disease. However, it is recommended that the high concentration of papaya extract will be used rather than the low and the medium. The results suggest that it may have a higher chance of healing relevant diseases since it had increased significantly the platelet count of the diseased mice. By means of bleeding time, the high concentration extract-treated groups showed no significant differences from the negative control. Treatment groups of low and medium concentrations did not significantly vary from the untreated mice, which manifested longer bleeding time than the negative control and high concentration treatment groups. Particularly, the high concentration extract induces short bleeding time which is similar to the negative control within two weeks.

3.2 Effect on Bleeding and Clotting time

The bleeding time method is widely used as general test to explore primary hemostasis (Colman *et. al.*, 1987). The most common use of this method is in place of preoperative screening potentially dangerous platelet disorders as stated by Edwin *et. al.* (2009). According to the American Hematology Society (2014), since it is prolonged in congenital or acquired platelet defects, the test has been also used to provide a screening for hemorrhagic tendencies from otherwise occult platelet disorders.

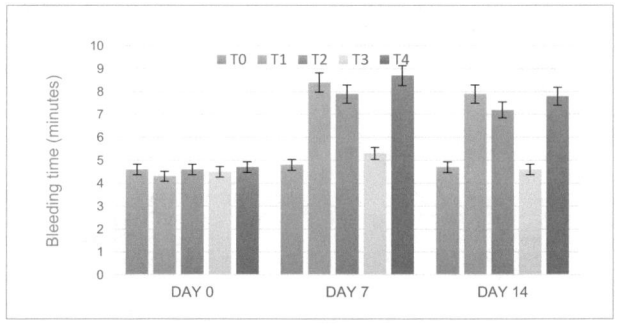

Figure 3. Bleeding time of mice at varying concentrations of *Carica papaya* fruit extract

By means of bleeding time as shown in Figure 3, the high concentration extract-treated groups showed no significant differences from the negative control. Treatment groups of low and medium did not significantly vary from the untreated mice, which manifested longer bleeding time than the negative control and high concentration treatment groups. Particularly, the high concentration extract induces short bleeding time, which is similar to the negative control within two weeks.

In terms of clotting time, results showed that it only took a week for all the treatments to shorten the clotting time as compared to the untreated group (Figure 4). However, low and medium concentrations were not as effective as the high concentration, because the two lower groups the manifested better results on the second week than during the first week.

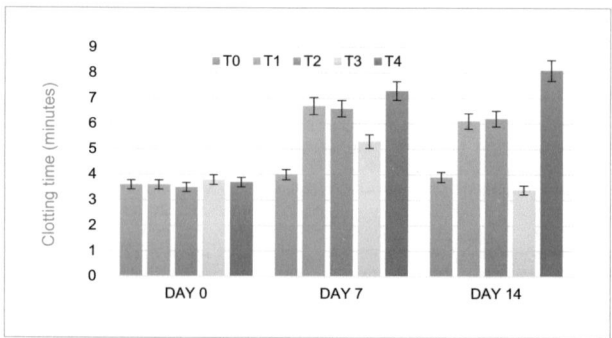

Figure 4. Clotting time of mice at varying concentrations of *Carica papaya* fruit extract

Results indicate that the high concentrated extract may possibly serve as an acceptable cure in the main effect of Dengue virus – lowered platelet count. Increasing number of blood platelets and consequently reduces the risk of having thrombocytopenia, and other related conditions such as bleeding that may lead to hemorrhage or Dengue Hemorrhagic Fever (DHF), which is known to be fatal. This curative action is assumed to be a direct effect of the extract on the hematopoietic systems. It is possible that the compounds found on the extract can interact and stimulate the formation and secretion of hematopoietic growth factors and committed stem cells. Specifically, stimulations of hematopoietic growth factors have been reported to enhance rapid synthesis of blood cells (Murray, 2009). *Carica papaya* leaf extracts is composed various phytochemicals like saponins, tannins and alkaloids, which are also found in the fruit, can act on the bone marrow to prevent its destruction and enhance its ability to produce blood platelets (Bhide *et. al.*, 2013). Moreover, these phytochemicals are also abundant in *Psidium guajava* leaves, which can also prevent platelet destruction in the blood and thereby increase the life of the platelet in circulation as supported by the study conducted by Uboh *et. al.* (2013).

3.3 Effect on RBC and WBC counts

Results reveal that Red blood cell count of mice differed significantly among treatments on the 7th day (p=0.012) but not during the 14th day (p=0.621). As shown in Figure 5, the number of RBC of mice treated with low, medium and high concentrations of papaya extract were significantly higher than the positive control mice, but comparatively similar with the negative control. Results indicate that on the second week of treatment, the extracts had no significant differences on the RBC count.

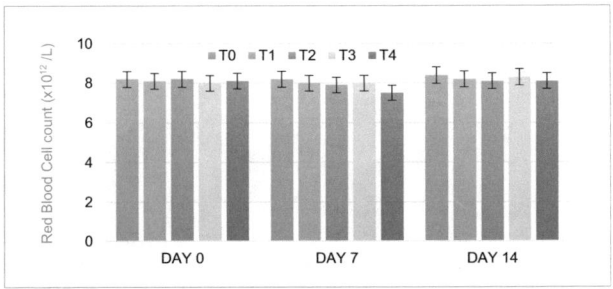

Figure 5. RBC count of mice at varying concentrations of *Carica papaya* fruit extract

ANOVA found that RBC count of mice differed significantly among treatments on the 7th day. Low, medium and high treatment groups showed significantly higher RBC counts than the positive control but not relatively similar with the negative control. On the other hand as graphed in Figure 6, ANOVA found no significant difference in the White blood cell count of mice among treatments on the 7th day (p=0.468) and 14th day (p=0.127). This means that the varying concentrations showed no significant effect on the WBC count having no manifested significant differences from the controls.

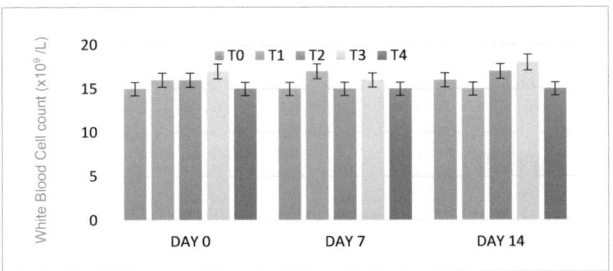

Figure 6. WBC count of mice at varying concentrations of *Carica papaya* fruit extract

3.4 Effect on Body Weight

The average weight of mice differed significantly among treatments on the 7th day and 14th day of treatment having p-values lesser than 5% level (Figure 7). Gain in weight was not significant during the 7th day (p=0.082) while a significant difference was found on the 14th day (p=0.000). Particularly that of the high concentration treatment group was nearly comparable to the weight of the negative control mice. Meanwhile, the diseased animals (positive control) manifested reduced weight.

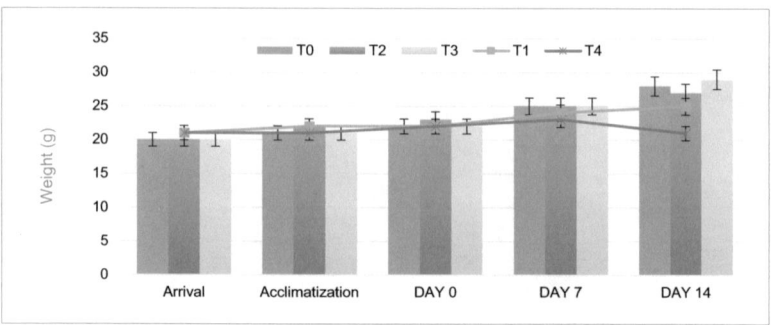

Figure 7. Body weights of mice at varying concentrations of *Carica papaya* fruit extract

One of the independent predictors of thrombocytopenia is decreased body weight as stressed on the study conducted by Cooper *et. al.* (2010). However, the results of the study on hand did not yield a relevant result in terms of body weight for the 7th day. Despite continuous treatment with varying papaya extracts concentration levels, platelet count consistently decreased in contrary with the increasing mice body weight for the same time being. On the other hand, results from day 14 concluded in favor to that conclusion of Cooper *et. al* (2010). Treatment groups of T1, T2 and T3 restored, or even succeeded their normal platelet levels which in correlation reflects to their increased body weight for day 14. Same trend was shown in terms of the T0 group, wherein an increase in weight was observed on day 7 in spite of significant loss in platelet count, with a subsequent and expected drop in weight corresponding to the continuously decreasing platelet count on the 14th day. Henceforth, the consistent body weight increase for these treatment groups may have been in line with the increase in food and water consumption similar to the study of Halim *et. al.* (2011).

4. CONCLUSIONS

The study was conducted to screen the thrombopoetic and hemostatic effect of Papaya (*Carica papaya* Linn.) fruit extracts on Aspirin induced-male ICR strain albino mice (*Mus musculus*), mimicking the adverse effect of Dengue fever, thrombocytopenia. The research dealt on different parameters namely: platelet counts, bleeding time, clotting time, number of red blood cells, white blood cells and body weight.

It is concluded, therefore, that Papaya, scientifically known as *Carica papaya*, fruit extract have significant thrombopoetic and hemostatic effect on the platelet counts, bleeding time and blood clotting time. Furthermore, the high concentration treatment was the most effective in exhibiting more evident changes in the experimental animals, including body weight.

It is in hopefulness of the researcher that the aforementioned findings in this present study be useful to the succeeding generations of researchers, working one definitive goal of improving the quality of health and life of humankind.

5. LITERATURES CITED

American Hematology Society (2014) *Blood*. Washington, DC.

Apostol, J., *et. al.* (2012) *Platelet-Increasing Effects of Euphorbia hirta Linn. in Ethanol-induced Thrombocytopenic Rat Models.* University of Sto. Tomas, Manila.

Bhide, R., *et. al.* (2013) Evaluation of Platelet Augmentation Activity of Carica papaya Leaf Aqueous Extract in Rats. Journal of Pharmacognosy and Phytochemistry.

Botting, RM., (2006). *The mechanism of action of Aspirin*. The William Harvey Research Institute.

Chaloob, A., *et. al.* (2009) *The effects of aspirin and fenugreek seed on the testes of white mice.* Fac Med

Colman R., *et. al.* (1987) Hemostasis and Thrombosis. Basic Principles and Clinical Practice. Philadelphia.

Cooper, HA., *et. al.* (2010) *Clinical implications of thrombocytopenia among patients undergoing intra-aortic balloon pump counterpulsation in the coronary care unit.* Georgetown University Hospital, Washington, DC

Gregg D. & Clermont PJ., (2003). *Cardiology patient page: Platelets and cardiovascular disease.* Circulation.

Halim SZ., *et. al.* (2011) *Acute toxicity study of Carica papaya Leaf extract in Sprague Dawley Rats.* Research gate.

Knowlton, K., *et, al.* (2009) *Mosquito-borne dengue fever threat spreading in the Americas.* Natural Resources Defense Council, New York.

Murray RK., *et. al.* (2000) *Red & White Blood Cells.* Harper's Biochemistry, McGraw-Hill, USA

World Health Organization (1997). *Dengue / dengue hemorrhagic fever.*